I0785423

Yoga Body

Quick yoga sessions you can do at home, Fast energizing yoga workouts, Yoga for a better night's sleep, Morning wake up routine, Yoga core workout, 20 minute cardio yoga workout,

By

Dee Persad

All Rights Reserved. No part of this publication may be reproduced in any form or by any means, including scanning, photocopying, or otherwise without prior written permission of the copyright holder.

Copyright © 2018

IF YOU ARE OVER 40 YEARS OLD, OR HAVE A HISTORY OF HEART DISEASE OR INJURIES, THEN YOU SHOULD BE MEDICALLY CLEARED BY YOUR PHYSICIAN BEFORE STARTING ANY EXERCISE PROGRAM.

Table of Contents

Introduction

Firstly I want to thank you for purchasing my book 'Yoga with Dee.'

Yoga is my passion and I wanted to distil the most effective Yoga techniques into a time-efficient results-driven set you can perform in your own home.

Many Yoga books have a great number of routines but their actual real-world applications are a little vague. I wanted specific routines to deliver specific results much like weight training back or biceps. But I wanted more than just muscle-stretching workouts. I wanted a Yoga routine for an energising wake up, toning core muscles, aiding restful sleep and many more. These techniques are designed to enhance your flexibility, build stamina, lose fat, tone muscles and give you a tremendous sense of well-being.

I have compiled the very best routines and yoga sequences to give you great results.

The routines duration will vary depending on the time you have, ranging from 5 minutes to 10, to 20 all working around your busy schedule.

For those of you more experienced Yogi's that want to get straight to the workouts please see the summary at the end of each routine for a quick easy go to option.

The key is to make the Yoga work for you!

1. Yoga Background

I wanted to give newcomers a little more info on the background of Yoga.

Yoga is a unique practice that connects the movement of the body and the fluctuations of the mind to the rhythm of our breath. Connecting the mind, body, and breath helps us to direct our attention inward. Through this process of inward attention. We become more aware of our experiences from moment to moment and through our movements. The awareness that we cultivate is what makes yoga a practice, rather than a task or a goal to be completed. Your body will most likely become much more flexible by doing yoga, and so will your mind.

This is not an overnight solution, and it will take time. Your body will need to adapt to the new fitness routines. This is completely normal. We will be focusing on keeping the body limber with flexibility exercise, and yoga. These exercises will help not only smooth your curves, but also coordinate your balance.

One of the best ways to keep fit is to keep mobile. If you can only do 10-20 minutes per session, that's fine too. Don't let time constraints or unrealistic goals be an obstacle, do what you can and don't worry about it. You will likely find that after a while your desire to practice expands naturally and you will find yourself doing more. With practice, focus and discipline your newfound agility will be balanced by strength, coordination, and will enhance your overall well-being.

2. Preparation

I always like to plan ahead when I'm going to do any Yoga, even if it's a case of quickly doing something before I head out to work.

Nutrition

Firstly, try not to eat a heavy meal 2 hours before exercise as it is likely we will be incorporating bending, stretching and floor work which your stomach will thank you for staying empty. If you feel that you need something to energise yourself before your workout then you can have small snacks such as nuts (high in protein) or half a glass of juice or protein shake to give you a kick-start up to 30 minutes before.

Prepare Your Workout Area

This is invaluable and makes so much difference - trust me! Be free of any distractions. So if you have just got home from work, leave your phone on silent in the kitchen, change clothes and get into the living room. If it's before work, get out of bed and get to the place where you will do your yoga and just begin. Don't stop to switch your phone on or check the news! These things will be automatic once you've done this a couple of times:

1. Put mobile phones on silent and ignore.

2. Turn Laptop, TV, Radio off if nearby.

3. Wear comfortable clothes.

You can use the floor or a Yoga mat to prevent slipping in the comfort of your own living room.

Remember whether you've got up 10 minutes early before work to do your yoga or you've allowed the entire Sunday morning - this is a part of the day that belongs to you and you alone. You mind must have no distractions to really benefit from the workouts.

3. 5 Minute Morning 'Wake Up' Routine

Even as little as 5 minutes of yoga each morning can help you get energised for the day ahead. Practicing yoga in the morning has many benefits. Not only is it the most peaceful time of the day without much distraction, it also helps you clear your mind, increase physical energy, endurance, and speed up your metabolism.

A) Mountain Pose

1. Stand with your feet together placed firmly on the ground.

2. Lift up through the crown of your head.

3. Round your shoulders and feel yourself lengthen up through all sides of your waist.

4. Breathe normally and focus.

5. Hold the pose and take 5 breaths in and out.

6. Although it may seem as though you are just standing there this pose promotes balance and directs your attention to the present moment where you are elongating your spine and preparing for the next pose.

The benefits: Improves posture and increases strength, power, and mobility in the feet, legs, and hips.

B) Tree Pose

1. Begin in the mountain pose.

2. Bend one knee, using your hand to bring your foot into the upper inner thigh. (Alternatively, bring the foot to the shin below the knee, or use the wall for balance.) Press into your standing foot, and lengthen up through the crown of your head.

3. Hold the pose and take 5-6 breaths here.

The benefits: This pose helps improve concentration and your ability to balance by strengthening the arches of the feet and the outer hips

C) Child's Pose

1. Transition to the floor and tuck your legs behind you in a kneeling position.

2. Reach up, breathe and lay your hands out in front of you walking them in front of you until you feel a stretch.

3. Breathe in your stretch here. Deep breaths inhaling and exhaling about 3-4 times.

4. If the poses are too much or you feel strain then child's pose is the one you can go to at any time. You can also use a towel to protect your knees if you feel any pressure or for additional support.

The benefits: This pose calms the body, mind and spirit. It gently stretches the low back, massages and tones the abdominal muscles. This pose also stimulates digestion and elimination of toxins from the body.

D) Cow pose

1. Transition from child's pose to cow pose.

2. Your shoulders should be stacked over your wrists and your hips over your knees.

3. Focus your gaze in between your hands. Don't forget to breathe!

4. Ensure equal weight is distributed through your body. Begin to relax your feet and engage your abdominal muscles which will begin to lengthen your spine.

5. Breathe in and out for 5 breaths.

The benefits: There are many physical benefits of Cow Pose, including toning the gastrointestinal tract and female reproductive system. It can also help to relieve stress from menstrual cramps, lower back pain, and sciatica.

E) Cat Pose

1. In this pose you feel like you are a puppet on a string where it pulls the middle of your back towards the ceiling.

2. Begin to press your hands and round your upper back. Drop your head, tuck your chin in toward your chest and your belly should move in towards your spine.

3. Breathe in and out 5 times.

The benefits: This Pose increases flexibility of the neck, shoulders, and spine.

F) Downward facing dog

1. Set the palm of your hands down onto the floor.

2. With your knees directly below your hips and your hands, slightly forward of your shoulders.

3. Tuck toes and lift hips up and back to lengthen your spine.

4. Exhale lifting your knees away from the floor and the heels are lifted. You should feel a good stretch in your hamstrings.

5. Breathe in and out 5 times.

Variation: (If you're inflexible keep your knees bent in order to bring your weight back into the legs.)

The benefits: A rejuvenating pose that energizes the body. This pose stretches the shoulders, hamstrings, calves, arches, and hands while strengthens the arms and legs.

G) *End of Practice: Child's Pose*

1. Finish the routine by bending your knees and returning to Child's Pose.

2. Breathe in here for 5 breaths.

3. Hold each pose and remember to breathe in and out 5 times in each position.

4. Summary: 5 Min Morning 'Wake Up' Yoga Routine

Here's a quick go-to summary of the exercises.

A) Mountain Pose
1. Hold the pose and take 5 breaths in and out.

B) Tree Pose
1. Hold the pose and take 5-6 breaths here.

C) Child's Pose
1. Breathe in your stretch here. Deep breaths inhaling and exhaling about 3-4 times.

D) Cow Pose
1. Breathe in and out for 5 breaths.

E) Cat Pose
1. Breathe in and out 5 times.

F) Downward facing dog
1. Breathe in and out 5 times.

G) Child's Pose
1. Breathe in your stretch here.
2. Deep breaths inhaling and exhaling about 3-4 times.

5. 10 Minute Morning 'Wake Up' Yoga Routine

Taking a peaceful moment for yourself at the start of each day will allow you to feel grounded re-charged, and in good spirits. This is the 10 minute version if you have more time to put into your workout.

A) Mountain Pose

1. Stand with your feet together placed firmly on the ground.

2. Lift up through the crown of your head.

3. Round your shoulders and feel yourself lengthen up through all sides of your waist.

4. Breathe normally and focus.

5. Hold the pose and take 5 breaths here.

6. Although it may seem as though you are just standing there this pose promotes balance and directs your attention to the present moment where you are elongating your spine and preparing for the next pose.

The benefits: Improves posture and increases strength, power, and mobility in the feet, legs, and hips.

B) Cow pose

1. Transition from child's pose to cow pose.

2. Your shoulders should be stacked over your wrists and your hips over your knees.

3. Focus your gaze in between your hands.

4. Don't forget to breathe!

5. Ensure equal weight is distributed through your body.

6. Begin to relax your feet and engage your abdominal muscles which will begin to lengthen your spine.

7. Hold pose for 5-6 breaths

The benefits: There are many physical benefits of Cow Pose, including toning the gastrointestinal tract and female reproductive system. It can also help to relieve stress from menstrual cramps, lower back pain, and sciatica.

C) Cat Pose

1. In this pose you feel like you are a puppet on a string where it pulls the middle of your back towards the ceiling.

2. Begin to press your hands and round your upper back. Drop your head, tuck your chin in toward your chest and your belly should move in towards your spine.

3. Hold pose for 5-6 breaths

The benefits: This Pose increases flexibility of the neck, shoulders, and spine.

D) Downward facing dog

1. Set the palm of your hands down onto the floor.

2. With your knees directly below your hips and your hands, slightly forward of your shoulders.

3. Tuck toes and lift hips up and back to lengthen your spine.

4. Exhale lifting your knees away from the floor and the heels are lifted. You should feel a good stretch in your hamstrings.

5. Breathe in and out 5 times.

Variation: (If you're inflexible keep your knees bent in order to bring your weight back into the legs.)

The benefits: A rejuvenating pose that energizes the body. This pose stretches the shoulders, hamstrings, calves, arches, and hands while strengthens the arms and legs.

E) Cobra

1. Spread your hands on the floor so they are placed under your shoulders.

2. Stretch your legs back so the tops of your feet are placed firmly into the floor.

3. Hug your elbows back and inhale.

4. Begin to straighten and lift your chest off the floor.

5. Hold the pose for about 15-30 seconds breathing easily.

6. Repeat the pose and breathe for a further 15-13 seconds.

7. Then release back on to Child's pose.

The benefits: Strengthens the muscles in the arms, shoulders and back. Also, helps to strengthen the spine, firm the buttocks and can help to relieve fatigue and stress.

F) Child's Pose

1. From Cobra Pose transition to the floor and tuck your legs behind you in a kneeling position.

2. Reach up, breathe and lay your hands out in front of you walking them in front of you until you feel a stretch.

3. Breathe in your stretch here. Deep breaths inhaling and exhaling about 3-4 times.

Variation: If the poses are too much or you feel strain child's pose is the one you can go to at any time. You can also use a towel to protect your knees if you feel any pressure or for additional support.

The benefits: This pose calms the body, mind and spirit. It gently stretches the low back, massages and tones the abdominal muscles. This pose also stimulates digestion and elimination of toxins from the body.

6. Summary: 10 Min Morning 'Wake Up' Yoga Routine

A) Mountain Pose
    1. Hold the pose and take 5 breaths here.

B) Cow Pose
    1. Hold pose for 5-6 breaths.

C) Cat Pose
    1. Hold pose for 5-6 breaths.

D) Downward Facing Dog
    1. Breathe in and out 5 times.

E) Cobra Pose
    1. Hold the pose for about 15-30 seconds breathing easily.
    2. Repeat the pose and breathe for a further 15-13 seconds.
    3. Release back into Child's Pose

7. 5 Minute Yoga Core Workout

There are individual yoga moves that you can follow to transition from one to the other or for specific needs you can concentrate on different areas.

I have a nice quick yoga session focusing on your abdominal muscles which has been very popular or start your day with a morning energising routine and wind down before bed in a session to relax your body and mind.

Let's go into detail about what we'll be doing.

This section will show you some techniques to help build core strength. Some studies have shown that yoga increases flexibility and reduces stress. Studies have shown after regular practice this help reduce belly fat and also reduces stress eating.

These postures will isolate your abdominal muscles and start to sculpt your abs. Start with our 5 minute Ab sequence and then move onto 10 minutes. A little everyday goes a long way to start burning belly fat and strengthen that core.

A) Tree Pose

1. Begin in the mountain pose.

2. Bend one knee, using your hand to bring your foot into the upper inner thigh. (Alternatively, bring the foot to the shin below the knee, or use the wall for balance.)

3. Press into your standing foot, and lengthen up through the crown of your head.

4. Take 5 deep breaths here and then change leg and repeat.

The benefits: This pose helps improve concentration and your ability to balance by strengthening the arches of the feet and the outer hips

B) Warrior Lunge Twist

1. Bring your hands into prayer pose.

2. Lunge forward with your left leg and bend your knee about 90 degrees, keeping your back leg straight.

3. Brace your abs in tight to your spine and rotate your upper body to the left.

4. Keep your spine long as you lean over your left leg and press your right elbow into the outside of your left leg.

5. Turn your head to look up toward the ceiling over your left shoulder.

6. Hold for 5 long, deep breaths and then untwist and return to standing. Repeat on the other

The benefits: This move engages your oblique's.

C) Extended Boat Pose

1. Sit on your hips with both legs extended in front of you.

2. Place your hands behind your hips and keep your back long as you lean back slightly and lift your legs off the floor, holding your tummy in and up the entire time.

3. Reach both arms out to the sides of your thighs. Lower your legs about 45 degrees, until your body resembles a wide 'V' shape.

4. Hold this position for 5-6 long, deep breaths (or up to 30 seconds).

Variation: Make it easier by bending your knees 90 degrees so your shins are parallel to the ground.

The benefits: This move builds core strength and endurance with this challenging, but very effective, pose. This can also help improve spinal stability.

D) Stacked Side Plank

1. Use your abdominals to stabilize your entire body as you balance on one arm and leg.

2. Lie on your right side with your knees straight. Place your right hand under your right shoulder.

3. Lift your hips off the floor until your body forms a straight line from your ankles to your shoulders.

4. Flex your feet and extend your left arm up to the ceiling. Breathe deeply for the duration of the exercise.

5. Hold this position for up to 30 seconds. Lower and repeat on the other side.

Variation: If this is too challenging, bend one (the bottom) or both knees to the floor to reduce the amount of weight that you have to lift.

The benefits: For this position use your abdominals to stabilize your entire body as you balance on one arm and leg. This move engages your core and strengthens the abdominal muscles.

8. Summary: 5 Minute Yoga for your Core

For those of you that already have knowledge of the yoga poses or for our experienced Yogi's, if you would like to go straight to the yoga routines without the explanations then the summary section at the end of each routine are for you.

A) Tree Pose
1. Take 5 deep breaths here
2. Change to opposite leg and repeat for 5 more breaths

B) Warrior Lunge Twist
1. Hold for 5 long, deep breaths and then untwist and return to standing.
2. Repeat on the other leg

C) Extended Boat Pose
1. Hold this position for 5-6 long, deep breaths (or up to 30 seconds).

D) Stacked Side Plank
1. Hold this position for up to 30 seconds.
2. Lower your leg and repeat on the other side.

9. 10 Minute Yoga Core Workout

This section increases what we did on our 5 minute yoga core section to a 10 minute sequence. The important thing is to concentrate on isolating those abs throughout and holding the postures. Don't forget to focus on your breathing. A Lot of the moves are similar however, we will be holding the postures for longer. As you begin to include these in your routine your abdominal area will feel stronger and more toned.

A) Mountain Pose

1. Stand with your feet together placed firmly on the ground.
2. Lift up through the crown of your head.
3. Round your shoulders and feel yourself lengthen up through all sides of your waist.
4. Breathe normally and focus.
5. Hold the pose and take 5 breaths here.
6. Although it may seem as though you are just standing there this pose promotes balance and directs your attention to the present moment where you are elongating your spine and preparing for the next pose.

The benefits: Improves posture and increases strength, power, and mobility in the feet, legs, and hips.

B) Tree Pose

1. Remain in the mountain pose.
2. Bend one knee, using your hand to bring your foot into the upper inner thigh. (Alternatively, bring the foot to the shin below the knee, or use the wall for balance.)
3. Press into your standing foot, and lengthen up through the crown of your head.
4. Take 10 deep breaths here and then change leg and repeat.

The benefits: This pose helps improve concentration and your ability to balance by strengthening the arches of the feet and the outer hips

C) *Warrior Lunge Twist*

1. Bring your hands into prayer pose.
2. Lunge forward with your left leg and bend your knee about 90 degrees, keeping your back leg straight.
3. Brace your abs in tight to your spine and rotate your upper body to the left.
4. Keep your spine long as you lean over your left leg and press your right elbow into the outside of your left leg.
5. Turn your head to look up toward the ceiling over your left shoulder.
6. Hold for 10 long, deep breaths and then untwist and return to standing.
7. Repeat on the other leg.

The benefits: This move engages your oblique's.

D) Extended Boat Pose

1. Sit on your hips with both legs extended in front of you.
2. Place your hands behind your hips and keep your back long.
3. As you lean back, slightly lift your legs off the floor, holding your tummy in and up the entire time.
4. Reach both arms out to the sides of your thighs.
5. Lower your legs about 45 degrees, until your body resembles a wide 'V' shape.
6. Hold this position for 10 long, deep breaths (or up to 60 seconds).

Variation: Make it easier by bending your knees 90 degrees so your shins are parallel to the ground.

The benefits: This move builds core strength and endurance with this challenging, but   very effective, pose. This can also help improve spinal stability.

E) Stacked Side Plank

1. Use your abdominals to stabilize your entire body as you balance on one arm and leg.
2. Lie on your right side with your knees straight. Place your right hand under your right shoulder.
3. Lift your hips off the floor until your body forms a straight line from your ankles to your shoulders.
4. Flex your feet and extend your left arm up to the ceiling. Breathe deeply for the duration of the exercise.
5. For this position use your abdominals to stabilize your entire body as you balance on one arm and leg.
6. Hold this position for up to 60 seconds. Lower and repeat on the other side.

Variation: If this is too challenging, bend one (the bottom) or both knees to the floor to reduce the amount of weight that you have to lift.

The benefits: This pose works your core, improves your arms, legs and wrist strength as well as improving your balance and concentration.

F) Bow Pose

1. Lie face down, then lift chest, arms, and legs off the floor.
2. Bend knees and reach back to grab outer ankles.
3. Lift your toes toward the ceiling, spin inner thighs in the same direction, and lengthen your tailbone toward the backs of your knees.

The benefits: This backbend stretches the whole front of the body, especially the chest and the fronts of your shoulders. It also massages your abdominal organs.

10. Summary: 10 minute Yoga Core Workout

A) Mountain Pose
1. Take 5 breaths here

B) Tree Pose
1. Take 5 deep breaths here
2. Change to opposite leg and repeat for 5 more breaths

C) Warrior Lunge Twist
1. Hold for 10 long, deep breaths and then untwist and return to standing.
2. Repeat on the other leg.

D) Extended Boat Pose
1. Hold this position for 10 long, deep breaths (or up to 60 seconds).

E) Stacked Side Plank
1. Hold this position for up to 60 seconds.
2. Lower leg and repeat on the other side.

F) Bow Pose
1. Hold for 30 seconds

11. 15-20 Minute Yoga Cardio Session

One of the great things about yoga is you can adapt the moves to the practice that you want. By adding more intensity to your workout you can increase your endurance and get that heart rate up!

Here are some yoga moves for a great cardio yoga session.

Try combining this with one of the 5 or 10 minute abdominal workouts for a full body workout.

A) The Plank

1. Starting with the plank is almost a workout on its own. If you are working out with a friend try challenging each other and see how long you can hold a plank for.
2. This move strengthens your core, tones your arms and glutes. Feel the burn!
3. Start with your body parallel to the Floor. The weight of the body is supported by straight arms and your toes.
4. Pull your abdomen up towards the spine tuck the pelvis in.
5. Your neck is a natural extension of the spine so keep the chin slightly tucked.
6. Keep your palms flat and elbows close to the side body. The joints are stacked with the wrists, elbows and shoulders in a straight line.
7. Your gaze should follow the spine and eyes are focused down.
8. Hold for 2-3 minutes.

The benefit: Increasing flexibility and great for core conditioning.

B) Plank Jacks

1. Hold a strong Plank Pose. When you're ready to start, hop both feet away from each other and then back together.
2. Keep your shoulders stacked over your wrists and engage your core throughout.
3. Repeat 10 times.

The benefit: The plank itself is a great exercise to develop core strength. By adding the jumping jacks movement you're turning this exercise into a great cardio workout that elevates your heart rate and burns even more calories.

C) Stacked Side Plank

1. Use your abdominals to stabilize your entire body as you balance on one arm and leg.
2. Lie on your right side with your knees straight. Place your right hand under your right shoulder.
3. Lift your hips off the floor until your body forms a straight line from your ankles to your shoulders.
4. Flex your feet and extend your left arm up to the ceiling. Breathe deeply for the duration of the exercise.

Hold this position for up to 60 seconds. Lower and repeat on the other side.

Variation: If this is too challenging, bend one or both knees to the floor to reduce the amount of weight that you have to lift.

The benefit: Planks work all the muscles you need to maintain proper posture including your shoulders, abs, chest, back and neck.

D) Mountain Climbers

1. From Plank Pose, draw your right knee to tap your right elbow. Bring your feet back together, and switch to tap your left knee to your left elbow.
2. Start at a nice slow and comfortable pace and either stay here or take it up a notch and quicken the pace to get that heart rate up!
3. Repeat 10 times first on the right knee and then on the left.

The benefit: This routine challenges your balance, agility, and coordination. Great for toning legs and abdominal area.

E) Crescent Lunge

1. The front foot of one leg remains grounded with the knee directly above and tracking the ankle in a 90 degree angle. The back leg is straight, no bend in the knee, and the weight is distributed backwards onto the toes.
2. Let your back heel push back and down towards the floor. Keep the pelvis tucked under with your ribcage lifted.   With your chin slightly tucked in.
3. The spine is long and extended. Keep your arms are straight with no bend in the elbows or the wrists. The hands can be together or separated and facing each other with the fingers spread wide. Gaze is natural and forward.
4. Hold and stretch for 2-3 minutes then swap legs.

Variation: If the High Lunge version is too difficult, or if you are warming up for your practice, do the Low Lunge version instead. Bring your back knee to the mat and un-tuck your back toes.

The benefits: A great standing pose that utilizes all the muscles in the body. This move is a dynamic standing yoga pose that utilizes and integrates the muscles in your entire body. It stretches and strengthens the lower and upper body, while creating stability and balance.

F) Lunge Jumps

1. Remain in the Crescent Lunge position with your right foot forward, then jump high to switch your feet so your left foot is forward.
2. Pause for just a moment before jump switching again.
3. Lunge 10 times and then swap sides.
4. The benefits: It strengthens and tones the thighs, hips, and butt, while the balancing aspect helps to develop flexible stability

G) Downward Dog Pose

1. Set the palm of your hands down onto the floor.
    With your knees directly below your hips and your
    hands, slightly forward of your shoulders.
2. Tuck toes and lift hips up and back to lengthen
    your spine.
3. Exhale lifting your knees away from the floor and
    the heels are lifted.

Variations: You should feel a good stretch in your
hamstrings. (If you're inflexible keep your knees bent in
order to bring your weight back into the legs.)

The benefits: One of the most iconic yoga poses that
requires good strength. This move can boost energy, aid
circulation, build upper body strength and increase
flexibility in the hamstrings.

H) Extended Boat Pose

1. This pose builds core strength and endurance. It may be challenging, but is very effective. This can also help improve spinal stability
2. Sit on your hips with both legs extended in front of you.
3. Place your hands behind your hips and keep your back long as you lean back slightly
4. Lift your legs off the floor, holding your tummy in and up the entire time.
5. Reach both arms out to the sides of your thighs. Lower your legs about 45 degrees, until your body resembles a wide 'V' shape.
6. Hold this position for 10 long, deep breaths (or up to 60 seconds).

Variation: If this is too difficult, try bending your knees at a 90 degree angle so that your shins are parallel to the ground.

The benefits: Helps build abdominal strength and endurance.

12. Summary: 15-20 Minute Yoga Cardio Session

A) The Plank

1. Hold for 2-3 minutes.

B) Plank Jacks

1. Repeat 10 times.

C) Stacked Side Plank

1. Hold this position for up to 60 seconds.

2. Lower and repeat on the other side.

D) Mountain Climbers

1. 10 times first on the right knee

2. Repeat on the left knee.

E) Crescent Lunge

1. Hold and stretch for 2-3 minutes.

2. Swap legs and repeat stretch.

F) Lunge Jumps

1. Lunge 10 times and then swap sides.

G) Downward facing dog

1. Breathe in and out 5 times.

H) Extended Boat Pose

1. Hold this position for 10 long, deep breaths (or up to 60 seconds).

13. Yoga Poses for Relaxation and a better Night's Sleep!

This is a great routine to help you relax before bed in 10-15 minutes. Remember to leave the stress of the day behind and focus on relaxation and breathing.

I would start your bedtime yoga routine with slightly stimulating poses and then slowly work your way to more restorative poses. Time to unwind!

A) Winding Down Twist

1. Sit cross-legged on the bedroom floor and exhale as you place your right hand on your left knee and left hand on the floor behind your tailbone.
2. Gently twist your torso to the left.
3. Hold for 2-3 Minutes.
4. Allow your gaze to follow, looking over your left shoulder. Breathe deeply, then return to center and repeat on opposite side.

B) Child's Pose

1. Sit up comfortably on your heels.
2. Roll your torso forward, bringing your forehead to rest on the bedroom floor in front of you.
3. Lower your chest as close to your knees as you comfortably can, extending your arms in front of you.
4. Hold the pose and breathe.
5. Breathe here for 3-5 Minutes.

Variation: At any time you feel the poses are too much or you feel strain child's pose is the one you can go to at any time. You can also use a towel to protect your knees if you feel any pressure or for additional support.

The benefits: This pose calms the body, mind and spirit. It gently stretches the low back, massages and tones the abdominal muscles. This pose also stimulates digestion and elimination of toxins from the body.

C) Bridge Pose

1. Lying on the floor bend your knees and set your feet on the floor, heels as close to your sitting bones as possible.
2. Exhale and press your inner feet and arms actively into the floor.
3. Begin to push your tailbone upward toward the pubis, firming the buttocks.
4. Lift the buttocks off the floor. Keeping your thighs and inner feet parallel.
5. Clasp your hands below your pelvis and extend through the arms to help you stay on the tops of your shoulders.
6. Lift your buttocks until the thighs are about parallel to the floor.
7. Keep your knees directly over the heels, but push them forward, away from the hips, and lengthen the tailbone toward the backs of the knees.
8. Lift the pubis toward the navel.
9. Lift your chin slightly away from the sternum and, firming the shoulder blades against your back, press the top of the sternum toward the chin.
10. Firm the outer arms, broaden the shoulder blades, and try to lift the space between them at the base of the neck up into the torso.
11. Stay in this pose and breathe for 1 Minute and release with an exhalation. Rolling your spine to the floor.

Variation: If you're flexible enough to tuck your shoulders under, you'll get an even greater heart opener.

The benefits: Bridge is a great bedtime yoga pose because it helps aid stress reduction and can improve your circulation.

D) Reclined Bound Angle Pose or Goddess Pose

1. Simply lie on your back, bring the soles of your feet together, and let your knees fall out to the side.
2. You can even prop your knees up with pillows if that makes the pose more comfortable.
3. Hold here for 15-20 breaths and then switch to the other side.

Variation: Just place a pillow under each knee for support. This is the perfect pose before transitioning to Corpse Pose.

The benefits: Reclined Bound Angle Pose will help you open up your inner thighs and hips.

14. Summary: Yoga Poses for relaxation and a better night's sleep

A) Winding Down Twist

1. Hold for 2-3 Minutes.

2. Breathe deeply, then return to center and repeat on opposite side.

B) Child's Pose

1. Breathe in your stretch here.
2. Deep breaths inhaling and exhaling about 3-4 times.

C) Bridge Pose

1. Stay in this pose and breathe for 1 Minutes and release with an exhalation. Rolling your spine to the floor.

D) Reclined Bound Angle Pose or Goddess Pose

1. Hold here for 15-20 breaths and then switch to the other side.

15. After Work 'Wind Down' Workout!

After an active day when you want to wind down and stretch out those aching muscles this is a great little routine to destress and relax your body and mind.

A) Mountain Pose

1. Stand with your feet together placed firmly on the ground.
2. Lift up through the crown of your head.
3. Round your shoulders and feel yourself lengthen up through all sides of your waist.
4. Breathe normally and focus.
5. Hold the pose and take 5 breaths here.

Although it may seem as though you are just standing there this pose promotes balance and directs your attention to the present moment where you are elongating your spine and preparing for the next pose.

The benefits: Improves posture and increases strength, power, and mobility in the feet, legs, and hips.

B) Downward facing dog

- Set the palm of your hands down onto the floor.

- With your knees directly below your hips and your hands, slightly forward of your shoulders.
- Tuck toes and lift hips up and back to lengthen your spine.
- Exhale lifting your knees away from the floor and the heels are lifted. You should feel a good stretch in your hamstrings.
- Breathe in and out 5 times.

Variation: (If you're inflexible keep your knees bent in order to bring your weight back into the legs.)

The benefits: A rejuvenating pose that energizes the body. This pose stretches the shoulders, hamstrings, calves, arches, and hands while strengthens the arms and legs.

C) Cobra Pose

1. Begin to transition to Cobra. Spread your hands on the floor so they are placed under your shoulders.
2. Stretch your legs back so the tops of your feet are placed firmly into the floor.
3. Hug your elbows back and inhale.
4. Begin to straighten and lift your chest off the floor.
5. Hold the pose for about 15-30 seconds breathing easily.
6. Repeat the pose and breathe for a further 15-13 seconds.

The benefits: Strengthens the muscles in the arms, shoulders and back. Also, helps to strengthen the spine, firm the buttocks and can help to relieve fatigue and stress.

D) Table Pose

1. Transition to all fours making sure your knees are directly under your hips.
2. Palms should be directly under the shoulders with fingers spread wide and facing forward.
3. Knees should be hip width apart and weight evenly distributed.
4. Engage the core muscles and keep back flat.
5. Breathe here for 3 breaths.

The benefits: This pose is designed to relax the spine and open the chest which helps you to breathe more deeply.

E) High Lunge

1. Step the right foot forward between your hands, with the knee directly over the ankle.
2. Tuck the back toes under and straighten the back leg.
3. Press your palms down and fingers or fists into the floor while lifting the crown of the head up towards the ceiling.
4. Roll your shoulders down and back and press the chest forward.
5. Your gaze should be straight ahead with the chin parallel to the floor.
6. Extend the back leg by pressing your heel towards the floor and by pressing the back of the knee up towards the ceiling.
7. Relax the hips and let them sink down towards the floor.
8. Breathe for 2-3 breaths.
9. Go back to Downward facing dog and repeat the pose stepping with left foot forward this time.
10. Return to Downward Facing Dog Pose.

The benefits: High lunge opens the hips and chest, stretches the groin and legs, lengthens the spine and strengthens the lower body.

F) Warrior 1

1. Start in Downward Facing Dog.
2. Step one foot forward between your hands.
3. Turn the back foot out approximately 45 degrees.
4. Line up heel to heel, or slightly wider.
5. Bend your front knee over front ankle while you stretch through
6. Inhale and lift your torso and arms up to the ceiling.
7. Breathe for 5-10 seconds

The benefits: This energizing pose strengthens your legs, arms, and back muscles. It also gives your chest, shoulders, neck, thighs, and ankles a great stretch.

G) Warrior 2

1. From Warrior 1, hinge forward at the hips and rest your abdomen on your front thigh, arms stay alongside ears.
2. Step back foot in and shift your weight into your front foot.
3. Lift your back thigh up and reach through back heel.
4. Spin inner back thigh up to the ceiling.
5. Press palms together and gaze forward at hands.
6. Hold Pose for 10 seconds.
7. Transition back to Downward facing dog.

Variation: Take arms alongside hips, or place hands on the floor or on blocks/towel under the shoulders.

The benefits: This pose strengthens your legs, outer hips, and upper back. It also helps improve balance and posture.

H) Pigeon Pose

1. Start the posture in Downward Facing Dog.
2. Bring your right shin forward, parallel to the front edge of your yoga mat as with the right knee toward right wrist and right ankle toward left wrist.
3. Extend your back leg behind you with toes tucked in
4. Reach your torso forward and down, and reach your arms long and in front of you.
5. Breathe in the stretch here for 10 seconds.
6. Repeat on the opposite leg and hold for a further 10 seconds.

Variation: When reaching forward you can bring your hands together as a pillow for your forehead, with your elbows out to either side.

The benefits: Helps to loosen up the hips.

I) Pleated Twist

1. Sit on the floor in a cross-legged position.
2. Elongate your spine, and as you inhale.
3. Place your right hand flat on the floor behind you and your left hand on your right knee.
4. As you exhale, move deeper into the twist while looking over your right shoulder.
5. Hold for five breaths, then switch sides.

Variation: If it's more comfortable, sit on a folded blanket to raise your hips.

The benefits: Twisting increases blood flow to the digestive organs, which is known to increase their ability to function.

J) Seated Forward Bend

1. Inhale lifting the arms over the head. Lift and lengthen up through the fingers.
2. Exhale and slowly lower your torso towards the legs.
3. Reach your hands towards the toes, feet or ankles.
4. Breathe in the stretch for 10 seconds.

Variation: For a deeper stretch use your arms to gently pull the head and torso closer to the legs. Press out through the heels and gently draw the toes towards you. Remember to breathe!

The benefits: Seated forward fold provides a deep stretch for the entire back side of body from the heels all the way to the neck.

16. Summary: After Work Wind Down Workout

A) Mountain Pose

1. Hold the pose and take 5 breaths here.

B) Downward Facing Dog

1. Breathe in and out 5 times.

C) Cobra Pose

1. Hold for 10 seconds.
2. Repeat the pose and breathe for a further 10 seconds.

D) Table Pose

1. Breathe here for 3 breaths.

E) High Lunge

1. Start on right leg.
2. Breathe for 2-3 breaths.

F) Downward Facing Dog
1. Breathe in and out 3-5 times.

G) High Lunge

1. Start on left leg.
2. Breathe for 2-3 breaths.
3. Transition back to Downward Facing Dog for 3 breaths.

G) Warrior 1

1. Breathe for 5-10 seconds.

H) Warrior 2

1. Hold Pose for 10 seconds.
2. Transition back to Downward facing dog for 3 breaths.

I) Pigeon Pose

1. Breathe in the stretch here for 10 seconds.
2. Repeat on the opposite leg and hold for a further 10 seconds.

J) Pleated Twist

1. Hold for five breaths, then switch sides.

K) Seated Forward Bend

1. Breathe in the stretch for 10 seconds.

17. 'One Exercise' Yoga Bedtime Pose

This is one of my favourite poses for getting a great nights sleep and it is one of the easiest! Have you ever felt like you wake up and don't feel like you've had a good night's sleep? The key is relaxing the body in the first place, winding down from the hustle and bustle and slowly cooling your mind for an amazing night's sleep.

A) Corpse Pose (Savasana)

1. Find a comfortable spot on the floor or you can do this one in bed.
2. Lie down facing upwards, separating your legs and letting your feet fall apart.
3. Close your eyes and feel your entire body begin to relax.
4. Lie here and breathe for 3-5 minutes. Feel your body begin to relax.
5. The benefits: This is also a great pose to relax your muscles and your mind. Ideally this is completed at the end of a yoga practice.

18. Conclusion: Final Notes

Thank for you purchasing my Book on yoga. There are lots of routines to choose from that you can do in the comfort of your home. We all know how difficult it is to fit in an exercise regime with hectic schedules. This book should help you find routines you can do easily from your home and even your bed depending on the intensity of the routine.

For those of you more experienced Yogi's that want to get straight to the workouts please see the summary at the end of each routine for a quick easy go to option.

I hope this book helps you reached your fitness goals depending on what you wish to achieve. By taking the first step of doing 5-10 minutes each day you will start to feel more relaxed, toned and flexible.

Begin to build on your routines and combine a cardio 15-20 minute session with a 5 or 10 minute abdominal routine depending on the time you have available.

There'll be hard times when you're tired or just want to chill, it's up to you to know when to push on and do that workout or just take a break. Even a 5 minute yoga session in the evening is better than nothing where you can unwind after a stressful day.

Try and keep to a schedule, keep working the muscles regularly and you will get results.

NAMASTE!

Dee

www.ingramcontent.com/pod-product-compliance
Lightning Source LLC
Chambersburg PA
CBHW070048260726
48658CB00002B/781